RoBBing Mind

Chuck Collins

Other works

Mystery Novels

The Radio Murders: The Collectors

The Radio Murders: The Caller

The Radio Murders: Barbicas (2014)

RoBBing

Mind

This book is dedicated to the men and women, families, professionals and scientists who work so hard to extend life and ease the suffering of brain cancer, stroke, traumatic brain injury and other things that can and <u>do</u> rob a mind.

The majority of the proceeds from the sale of this publication will <u>always</u> go toward aiding their efforts.

RoBBing Mind by Chuck Collins

This book is owned by Chuck Collins, Studio D Books and principally edited by Pat Fernberg with help from Lou Lange
Cover Illustration Copyright © 2013 by Chuck Collins
ISBN-10: 0615892248
ISBN-13: 978-0615892245
Cover photograph by Lenora Enking
Cover design by Chuck Collins, Studio D Books
Author photograph by James Smith.

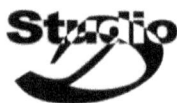

For Monika,

I will love you always

"You think you're Iron Man, but you're not."

~E.C. "Al" Collins

RoBBing Mind

Restless Machine

In 2007 a 67 year old man woke in his south Arlington area home (Akron, Ohio). It was a typical Tuesday morning. He was not feeling particularly well and mumbled something about a stomach ache to his wife. He even vomited, a rare occurrence and was feeling flu-like symptoms. But Mr. K was of strong Hungarian stock and it was a workday so preparing for work was his immediate concern.

He ignored the slight blur in his vision, often closing one eye to navigate the usually heavy expressway traffic and continued to attribute the fogginess to poor food choices the night before.

Mr. K, the shift supervisor, arrived at work right on time. He was always on time. But this morning something was not quite right. Mr. K had a far-off look in his eyes and when asked about the day's jobs he could not find the words to describe the duties on the schedule, neither could he remember any of the men's names nor what to call coffee or the materials he used every day.

Mr. K's alarmed coworkers called emergency services. It was quickly discovered that the otherwise healthy man had suffered a massive stoke and was only minutes away from a deadly serious neurological event.

9

But the blockage was slow enough for the brain to continue functioning as it had day in and day out for so many years.

Mr. K's experience is just one example of the power of the brain and it is not as rare as you might think. He was admitted to Summa Akron City hospital and through extensive treatment and rehabilitation he is now fully recovered in spite of the fact that the stroke affected critical sections of his brain.

Even under extreme stress or massive trauma there seems to be a resiliency, sometimes called a plasticity whereby the brain uses every last possible tool at its disposal to continue doing what is was designed to do: to keep us living, not just alive, but living.

In the annals and lore of law enforcement there are examples of someone with severe brain injury appearing to follow daily routines even as the rest of the body shuts down and death is eminent.

The human brain is a miracle. And that is the approach I will take in sharing these experiences with you. While there are hundreds of thousands of volumes – scholarly and otherwise - written by highly qualified scientists and others on the working of the brain, this is a personal accounting from a very intimate point of view. This is what could happen, the choices one must make, when one is faced with events that rob a mind.

RoBBing Mind

Introduction

How can a good attitude, good genes and good luck help prevent a fate worse than death?

What an audacious statement! What could be a fate worse than death, and how can we possibly control such a harsh reality?

My friend Dr. Terry Gordon can tell you what a fate worse than death is, as can my long-time friend Dr. Daniel Steinberg PhD. It might be robbing a young man, Terry's son, of all of life's joys and leaving him imprisoned in a broken body, justifiably bitter and feeling contempt for life although clinging to it as we all might. In his book *No Storm Lasts Forever*, Terry tells of his journey and the secrets hidden in plain sight for us, free of charge.

With Dan it is the loss of his child, Elena, just as she was entering her own brilliant light, days from her 7th birthday. Elena succumbed to an illness that is as ruthless as it is unpredictable. Dan and his wife spread their pain as thinly as possible relying on a gracious community of friends and colleagues as well as their surviving daughter to "love them through the darkness." You can learn more about this amazing man and a thousand other things he teaches at his

13

excellent website dimsumthinking.com.

In my case the 'fate worse than death' would be the erasure of my ability to communicate orally and in writing, my intellect and the very thing my family loves about me. It would have been robbing my mind.

In these pages I chronicle almost from the start the process and choices made to take a bad situation and turn it into the best possible scenario, not only for me and my family, but hundreds of thousands of people who might find themselves in similar straits. This book is not just for sufferers of brain tumors, but for stroke victims and those with externally caused brain trauma. This is for you; this is for us.

In the spring of 2013, I began having odd sensations on the left side of my body. I had turned 60 that year and things happen – or so I told myself. At just over 6 feet tall and carrying around 50 more pounds than was prudent, I had begun a calorie reduction program the previous fall and had lost about 30 pounds. I still had a long way to go.

Work had become more detailed and my 2009 Toshiba laptop had become almost an appendage. From upper management and programming duties for Rubber City Radio Group in Akron, Ohio, editing images and audio for radio to writing novels to managing the station's social media initiatives, I was sitting a lot and getting little exercise above the elbows!

My wife, Monika, whom you'll read about quite a bit in this observation, was after me to exercise more, but that mostly went unheard.

My blood pressure had started a slow rise. It had been a point of pride that I maintained a healthy BP while almost all the men in my extended family of my generation had to struggle with hypertension. Not unusual for African-American males. Those two little numbers, my blood pressure, soon played a pivotal role in discovering a frightening reality.

What happened next still astonishes me, but as the result of the work of some fine scientists and medical professionals, I am here to tell the story, and my intentions are to help you pay closer attention and possibly avoid a mind destroying fate, the possibility of which still haunts me.

It is also important for me to explain that the majority of the proceeds generated by this story will go directly to further research on brain health and cancer prevention, and to help families facing such challenges. Giving back is an imperative because I have been allowed to keep everything I have – and so much more.

Thank you for reading my story!

RoBBing Mind

The numbers are hardly conclusive, but according to the National Cancer Institute part of the National Institute of Health, in the course of a year 160,000 to 180,000 Americans are diagnosed with some form of brain tumor. Of these patients around 30,000 of these are tumors that originate in the brain or primary brain tumors and are considered cancerous. In about a third of those diagnosed the tumor can present a particularly aggressive nature making it difficult to eradicate, control, predict or even treat. These are figures reported by larger institutions and it is believed by many that the numbers are understated.

While specific data is also wide ranging, what is startling about these figures is that the survival rate for the most common of these tumors remains well below 50% and even the doctors who have devoted their careers and their lives to this disease still consider it incurable.

This is the story of one member of a club no one ever asked to join and from which there is no resignation. A club that includes prominent names such as Film Critic Gene Siskel, Sens. Arlen Specter and Ted Kennedy, Entertainers George Harrison and

17

Lou Rawls, baseball great Gary Carter and many more. It is a club that once offered few options but in time and with the advancement of science, positive outlooks are becoming more frequent. As you will see, while medicine is important, the real game-changer starts with something we all can control: our attitude.

Reader's note: The first 6 chapters were created as an immediate blog and recorded almost as it happened in the spring and summer of 2013.

July 16, 2013, about 4pm

1 - The Beginning.

Maria's eyes were like twin moons circling Planet Fear, my new home world. Her left eye belonged to the scientist, strong and confident; the right eye belonged to the woman, astonishingly sympathetic. Both eyes watched and waited for their time to shine into the night I was entering. Maria knew it was going to be a difficult message to deliver, but she had done so, or something very much like it, for more years than her youthful face showed.

"We found something…suspicious."

Really, I thought, *suspicious*? For the last dozen years part of my life as a mystery novelist had been steeped in finding the suspicious and making it fun, exciting and enticing. Mystery fiction lives in the colorless corners of human fear and desperation. In creating those spaces one must try to understand the impact. Until that afternoon I had no idea what the product I was trafficking was really like.

The face of Dr. Maria C., "just Maria, I hate titles," had harmonious features, just enough to support those big hazel eyes. Her hair was pulled back tightly, adding to the efficiency of the professional. But her smile was easy and fluid. She wore minimal makeup. I detected no scent from her whatever.

Maria, at about 5 foot 4 inches, commanded the room. Nothing else was more important than me and her message. I will have similar encounters with different doctors, nurses and others over the next few months. I have yet to become accustomed to the impact.

What brought me to the ER that beautiful summer day really started back in March of that year, very close to the 35th anniversary of our first marriage, Monika and me. March 5th is more than a number on a calendar under normal circumstances. But what happened next has added new weight to that date forever.

I was standing in my little studio, Studio D, where I do most of my air work. Visiting at that moment was someone I have known longer than 40 years, Phil Levine, one of the account executives at WAKR/WONE. He and I were just talking about radio business and a little bit about life. Suddenly, quite suddenly, the left side of my body seemed to spring a leak and lost 80% of its communication with central control, with my mind.

This part is still difficult to explain. Imagine half of your body "going to sleep," much like sitting on your leg in just that way, or having your arm in an odd position for longer than you should. Once you bring things back to normal there is that time when feelings are coming back but not quite and not quite fast enough. I have always found it uncomfortable and perhaps the worst part of the experience. This was like that on a much grander scale.

There was more. The feeling seemed to extend from my left leg and arm into my left trunk just enough to know it was an entirely new sensation. Along with that came a sense of unease that while this was neither weakening me, nor causing loss of balance nor even pain something brand new had occurred.

Because of that sensation alone I told my fiend Phil to stand by, that I might need help.

My first thought was that I was experiencing a stroke, for me one of the most feared attacks and something that I saw close up and while very young, perhaps age 8.

It was what I still remember as the lessons of Uncle Charlie. I was named after my father's older brother, Charles Arthur Collins. Yet my most vivid memory of Uncle Charlie is after he had a stroke. He was in his early 50's and it was a debilitating, face melting, gait robbing event from which he never really recovered.

I was at just the right age for that event to have a profound impact. I became aware of probably one of the cruelest of the many cardiovascular/neurological diseases. On that day in Studio D, standing there with Phil able to help if needed, I knew what to check to determine whether I was having a stroke.

I ticked off only one of six on my list. My speech was not slurred. I could see equally well out of both eyes and although the tingling remained on my left side, I told Phil I was fine, he could go on about his business. I had no problem getting back to my office and in a few minutes got back to work. I did no follow-up. Sadly, I believe that is how most men would have handled the event. "I'm fine."

I was not fine.

That weekend it happened again. Part of what I do is host crowds of people at community events, although it can make for a long night it is very enjoyable. The first 6 hours of the Catholic Charities Community Services Summit County Monte Carlo Night went very well. Then, as I was reading off winning numbers and names at the prize drawing conclusion of the evening that strange out-of-control feeling returned. Again the left side of my body began tingling with that better than half-way asleep, numbing sensation. Only our WAKR/WONE sales manager Dominic Rizzo noticed the look of concern on my face. Dom was helping with the drawing. He reads people well, it is one of the things that makes him a good sales person. And Dom knew me well and while there were no symptoms anyone would see, only the ones I felt, he knew something was not right.

After sitting a bit and drinking a little water I completed the event, but the disturbing sensation lasted the whole night and all the next day with more profound numbness. At this point any reasonable person would have headed to the ER, or at least have made an immediate appointment with a doctor.

Not me. I shook it off, but the symptoms

came back, several times in fact with new components like a spoiled child asserting himself with increasing insistence. Soon odd sensations in my taste buds and saliva flow accompanied the events, as I called them. I would recognize these little visitors, wait until they passed and be thankful when nothing bigger happened, such as passing out, losing the use of my limbs or experiencing other stroke symptoms. Nothing bigger did happen but the symptoms did not go away entirely. I was playing with fire and I knew it.

Now you know a little about this mule-headed man. What surprised me is how easy it was to remain in denial about my own health and events that were clearly out of the ordinary.

As we continue this journey you will see that it all fit a pattern that has shaped my life. And I am certain that either you know someone very much like me, or you may be guilty yourself.

Thankfully there are moments that one can't ignore and people who come into our lives with a power to change the course we are on. I believe we get into trouble when we fight these energies, and I believe that they are greater than anything else in life.

While these numbing episodes continued for four months and other things occupied my time they refused to move to the background of a busy life.

That is until Dr. Terry Gordon, perhaps unwittingly intervened.

One fine June day I was sitting in the beautiful backyard of Terry's home. Dr. Gordon had become something of a legend in our area, not only because of his immense skills as a cardiologist (now retired), innovator and community supporter, but because of the tragedies that had marred his otherwise rich life and how he came to handle these crushing turns of fate.

Terry and I became friends for several reasons but one was a love for books and writing. He has written a bestselling memoir, *No Storm Lasts Forever* detailing his journey and so much more. He had asked that I come over because he had written a novel and wanted my input.

To this day I'm not sure why I decided to tell Terry about the symptoms I had been experiencing. In fact there were several moments when I wanted to cancel the visit, but fate intervened and it was *just to be*.

Terry listened to my story and almost immediately retrieved a cuff and stethoscope from his home and took my blood pressure. It was extremely high (202/109). He insisted that I see a doctor right away.

That set me on a journey toward treating my hypertension. The events, it was believed, were trans ischemic attacks, TIA's or mini strokes.

With low-dose medication my blood pressure was under control which even surprised my doctor and the larger numbness events seemed to subside. But now there were smaller, more frequent events, about three a day. Both Terry and my doctor remained concerned, so was I.

But rationalization came easily for me. I blamed everything from a pinched nerve to the way I slept to my laptop searing nerves in my thigh. Yet there came a point when I knew something was still wrong and I as beginning to suspect that it was not so simple.

My doctor, also concerned that the events may be neurological in origin, set me up for two scans. One was not easy to get and I would have had to wait three weeks. Again the inner debate raged. But I had been worn down and by then I was frightened.

I was not going to wait three weeks. I was not going to wait one more day. I drove to the ER in Cuyahoga Falls still feeling that I was wasting everyone's time, not to mention spending deductible money that we didn't have. But it was now the business of finding out what was wrong and getting better and at that moment there was no price tag.

We have come full circle, from the moment in March when things seemed to change to entering the Summa Health Care system in my town of Akron, Ohio on July 16, 2013.

I have since learned that Maria, Dr. C was a resident and had not talked to my kind of patient often. She told me that, in preparation for delivering the news, she had imagined how she would tell a family member that CT scans had exposed a mass in his or her brain – *in my brain.*

I remember reading about reactions to that kind of bad news – news that still held a lot of uncertainty. Most write of anger and denial, fear, bargaining and more before acceptance and determination to beat the beast, your basic seven stages of grief. I didn't have any of that at that moment.

What I had was an incredible sense of wonder. I wondered what this really meant. I wondered if it was going to compromise my head, my personality and my ability to do what I am doing right now: writing. If the latter becomes reality, then, as one of my favorite characters in my novel *The Radio Murders: The Collectors* exclaims, "I mays well just go on up to Jesus right now."

But here is the odd part: the tumor is shared across the right parietal and temporal lobes of my brain, in a section that is partially responsible for the motor functions, sensory sensations of the left side of my body and some unknown (to me) temporal lobe functions. And as I write this it has not yet affected my speech, vision or reasoning. In the words of a physician's assistant from neurosurgery, if you're going to have a brain tumor and you are right handed, it's best to have it in the right side of the brain. Of course, I'd rather not have it at all.

As part of my recovery and ultimately my journey, I began keeping this running account of my feelings, observations and a little about the people I have met along the way. It had become a combination of game and test. Remembering names and engaging the caregivers is important under the best of circumstances. In this case it had become an obsession. I tried to assign face, job and name to virtually everyone with whom I had contact, from surgeons to housekeeping, nurses, transporters and everyone who worked so hard to care for patients like me.

My brain team started to form. First there was Shannon the neurosurgery physicians' assistant, an energetic red-head who knew how to defuse words like 'tumor' and 'cancer.' She laid out the plan for how we were going to discover "clues" and tackle the problem one step at a time. Then there was Brittany, thin and blonde, the neurology physicians' assistant had intense eyes and a fast-paced way of talking that she could stop on a dime to hear what Monika or I had to say.

Right behind her was Ryan, Dr. L. a big man with a "go ahead, try and shake me" kind of face who had an air of–the only way I can put it–*this is what we have and this is how we're going to beat it.* He reminded me of a former NFL player who came back to teach high school football, except that he was neither.

One last person I want to add is my new Internal Medicine doctor. Dr. Kim M was pretty and youthful for her nearly 50 years, brunette hair cresting below her shoulders. She actually glowed with confidence like most moms of boys (3 of her 5 are boys). That assuredness did not radiate *from* her necessarily, rather was projected into me, Monika and the process. There was not a doubt in her mind that we would come out of this better!

And what about Monika? That is the real story as you can imagine. In many ways she has had the toughest job.

In a hospital setting time has a way of fragmenting. For the patient, especially a surgical patient, it flows with huge gaps of unconsciousness and we are generally comfortable and cared for. For families there is little reprieve. The clock slows and the anticipation of news, good or bad, shadows every moment with anxiety. While there is discomfort, pain and possibly danger in treatment for the patient, it is the families who must endure in a very real way, the reality of any medical crisis.

And it is that reason that much of this story will focus on Monika and the families of other patients. You are the ones who must find courage, hope and strength.

2 - Magnetic Personality

When does one become comfortable with the word "cancer?" I'm convinced that it is only when checking horoscopes.

Through my entire life "cancer" has meant a death sentence, the beginning of the end, and worse, a stark illustration of how your bad habits had finally caught up with you.

Mom had five brothers and sisters and while she remained cancer-free for all her 92 years, every one of her siblings had cancer and all but one died of it. Mom was the eldest and except for her baby sister, a child born when my mom was 13, they all died before she. They had lung cancer, breast cancer, uterine cancer and one uncle actually had cancer of the heart's pericardial sac that was discovered after his heart finally failed.

Smoking, drinking, smoking and drinking, living with someone who smoked and drank—it always seems to come down to the stuff we do. My tumor is suspiciously like those some alarmists attribute to cell phone use, something I have done since the early 90's. I call them alarmist now, but who knows, I may call

31

them prophets tomorrow.

As the investigation began and grew more intensive, my friend Terry Gordon had a suggestion when I did have to deal with the confinement of the MRI machine, "close your eyes before they roll you in and keep them closed." He was right. When the time came I had the Brandenburg Concerto (Bach) serenading me through thick headphones, kept my eyes closed and the notoriously confining and noisy diagnostic tool was not so unpleasant.

I had to use the occasion to ask the MRI tech about the possibilities of using a $5 million machine as a murder weapon. (ABW, that's my motto: *Always be Writing*). It turns out a scene I was working on in my latest novel featured an MRI as a source of fear, torture and even death. Mike, the tech, gave me some good ideas, especially for one of the final scenes in which a particular nasty assassin gets his due.

The digital salami slicer caught a pretty good look at the little monster, as Monika calls it. Imagine three unequal disks of errant tissue about the size of Eisenhower silver dollars joined concentrically by a third and just nesting in the region of my right temporal and parietal lobes. Armed with these images the neurosurgeons got me on the OR schedule just a day and a half later. Of course, as with any procedure dealing with a major organ there are potential dangers.

The greatest of which is the tumor having a deeper grip on my gray matter and a possibility of a return engagement. That will all come out in the lab. They told me that they might get results on the composition of the mass before they closed me up. By this time tomorrow (2:45pm EDT July 19, 2013) I would have a pretty good picture of my immediate future. As long as I can talk and write (reasonably intelligently) I can deal with almost anything.

Monika and I along with my best friend Keith decided do a little head shave just to save the physician's assistant the trouble.

Before going to much further, I have to write a little more about Monika. It is no secret among those treating the seriously ill that the greater burden falls on the ones closest to the patient. In the case of my wife, Monika is my rock, although she will quickly tell you that I credit her with way too much strength. That day she was probably two words away from tears at any given minute. But as they say, courage is not the absence of fear, but the way we handle it.

Monika is handling this entire adventure better than most people could. How do I know this? Were the situations reversed, I would be a quivering mass. She is the best person for me, no matter what life throws at us. There needs to be a stronger word than "love" for how I feel about my wife.

3 - Bringing the Pain

As I write this I am about 14 hours out of surgery. The good news is that all went well. The bad news is that the spot where they installed a *switch plate* hurts like the dickens. Finding myself in the ICU I was stepping down from a very traumatic event. Some of the names I need to acknowledge are Melissa, Denise, Michelle, Tina and James, all nurses caring for patients at varying levels of post-op and intensive care. They helped me through my first night. And damn are they good at what they do!

Tina did an amazing thing for me. In the night I had two awful reactions, one was from morphine, the other was my first panic attack. I was in pain and my blood pressure would not stabilize. Denise had no choice but to control the pain so that I would relax. Eventually I was out of the dark, thanks to her. But Tina came in later and did something that went beyond the science of nursing and illustrated the innate ability to understand the person. I needed rest, not stimulation, but I believe she understood that rest for me might involve something more than just quiet. I asked her for my iPhone so I could listen to the podcasts that usually guide me off to sleep. The device's battery had drained and she rooted through my heavy backpack to find the power cord and in 10 minutes I was listening to weird radio: The **Phil Hendrie Show** and **Coast to Coast AM** with **George Noory**. Not that these programs put me to sleep, on the contrary they entertain even as I drift off.

I'm not sure if I would know Tina's face but I will never forget what she did for me that night. This may seem like a small thing, but it was common among the nurses at Summa and I was truly inspired.

There came a time during the day when I needed a gentle drill sergeant. That was James, right on time. He could see that I was improving rapidly and needed to get on my feet. James understood my discomfort from a man's point of view, for example the sooner the Foley catheter came out the better. He was fun and frank. We were up and about in probably record time. I was only one full day in ICU before getting out and in my hospital room. James and the rest of the staff in ICU had a great deal of understanding about the science of post-op procedures, but they start their work from an even deeper understanding of important human needs. That is not easy. But they do it. I will never forget the care I received in those critical 24 hours after a major surgical procedure. In the course of this surgical part of my recovery (something that will extend into nearly the remainder of the summer, although I didn't know it at the time), I will encounter two-dozen such caregivers and to a man and woman they all displayed the same compassion.

I also have to thank Tony and Diane Agnesi. They are simply amazing people. They sat with Monika while she waited to hear the news, good or bad, from my surgeons. It was not just the companionship; it was the way in which they embraced my frightened wife. It takes a strong faith and wisdom to do what Tony and Diane did that day. They don't just do this for people they consider friends, they are the rare couple who have enough love to share with a whomever needs it. Tony (Nick Anthony) and Diane take each day and try to make it better for someone, and in doing so make it a better world little by little.

Nick and I go back more than 25 years. He was one broadcaster who gave me a chance to prove myself within 16 months of getting sober in 1986. I will write more about that in the coming pages. But it is important to note here that while it was a risk, Nick always sees the best in me, even if I don't see it myself. Through trust, frank discussions and support he has not only made me a better broadcaster and a better writer, but a better person.

If I live to be 100 I can never thank him enough.

4 - A Study in Contrast.

Things began moving quickly. I was released from the ICU hours faster than most people thought possible. Not that I was rushing things, but the best place to recover from something like this ordeal has to be at home.

Welcome to Howard's world (not his real name). My first roommate since being admitted had a massive stroke in exactly the wrong place: the left frontal lobe. Howard was having trouble remembering what to call the light over his bed and had forgotten his wife's name.

Nursing Student Danielle and an RN named Ellen helped him get up in bed, and techs Stephanie and Christopher figured out his spoken code for turning off the TV.

Nursing assistant Dawn said I reminded her of Denzel Washington (I *don't* look like Denzel). I told her she reminded me of Ellen Barkin. We were even.

Day Three brought terrible waking dreams. I considered the realization that I was no longer the same person, that I must identify with the event that has occurred, a situation that less than a generation ago would have had a dramatically different, and quickly progressing fatal outcome. Modern nuclear medicine, magnetic imaging and a host of other inventions and innovations have given these talented men and women on my surgical team the ability to go into a man's brain and remove damaging tissue. That is not to say it is easy or simple, but it is done every day.

At this point in my journey I had no idea how deeply into those innovations I would still travel and how profoundly they would affect my prognosis.

Science is fact, often cold and unforgiving, but the real miracle is the way I have been treated by these caring individuals. These are times that can block the sun, if we let them. The medical team and all my caregivers, along with my family and friends were not going to let that happen. Neither was I.

A picture of me at that moment would look like I had gone three rounds with Mike Tyson. Swelling from the surgery had startling consequences including my greatest concern: an inability to speak clearly. I had been told that I was neurologically intact (no small achievement given the circumstances), but I was still worried about sounding like my Uncle Charlie!

Granted, it was more than vanity that fueled my concern; it was—and is—a nearly 40 year career that could quickly end with a condition known as *dysarthria*. You will read more about that as I move from relative health to stark terror to being a new person known as a brain tumor, cancer survivor.

The central focus of this book, indeed the only reason I am writing it, is to support families who are dealing with this devastating condition. What it is not is an attempt to add to the vast knowledge base of brain science and medicine.

This is about the human experience and I can't stress that enough.

We still know so little about the human mind. Yet in some respects it is the pin that links us all. Scientists are quickly learning more about the mechanics and anatomy of the brain. But with every answer comes more questions. So it is the families and loved ones of a person dealing with a compromised mind who are often shattered by the daily challenges and while hospitals such as Summa offer excellent resources in support, the ones who need it most may be the last to take advantage of the programs.

I was constantly reminded of this when I started paying attention to the activities on this hospital floor devoted primarily to neurology.

The greatest lesson came from observing the visitors. Coming to the hospital to visit is boring, uncomfortable and the patient is at his or her worst. But when you are on the other side, when you are the patient, those visits are very important. I mentioned my roommate Howard who had expressive aphasia – the inability to communicate what he means. Howard had asked to see his wife many times and she had yet to visit. Monika was very careful not to express how devoted she and I are to each other, not wanting him to feel even more lonesome. She is thoughtful like that. But she never missed an opportunity to make eye contact with him, listen to what he had to say even though it was difficult to understand. Howard would always end these brief encounters with, "thank you, sweetheart," and a broad smile. For a moment he was not so frightened.

On the floor, and throughout this experience, you can see a wide range of responses from family. There were more men than women admitted and there are reasons for that. Wives wore worried looks framed with fear that they tried to hide. It is almost impossible to hide the impact of the gravity of these changes, especially in the case of strokes.

Another thing you notice in a hospital setting such as Summa are the stories that continue just beneath the surface. Twice that afternoon there were pages for "OR team to emergency!" The mystery writer in me immediately went to gun shots or very bad auto accidents.

This is a Level One Trauma center and people

find themselves here as they face the very last hope to survive the unimaginable. A brain trauma such as mine also gives one reason to make assessments about life and death. I had a small stack of silver dollar-sized glop in the most important part of my body, perhaps short of the heart. I was healing nicely yet I could not help wondering what happened in that emergency room. I hoped those surgeons did their best work that night and every night.

It became a necessary diversion because somewhere in this experience there were mounting signals, messages that this adventure was about to become very different and very dangerous.

5 - A Fortnight With Mahesh

Doctors are, by design, the most analytical people in the world. As such they must calibrate their communications to the understanding of the patient. When talking to me, oncologist Dr. S. Mahesh started from the start and we quickly established that I knew what had happened and had a pretty good idea what I was facing. Still, he had to talk to a man about the possibility of having brain cancer. That had not occurred to me until I was surrounded by the oncology team, even with cancer there are degrees, levels and widely ranging outcomes.

The signals were becoming clear and it was a fast blast back to Planet Fear: this was no simple tumor, degaussing and extraction.

Dr. Mahesh and I did establish a rapport and he was able to understand the things that were important to me and how we could fit the treatment options into my life, as I live it now. He used language, such as taking about two weeks as *a fortnight*.

"I said that because you are a writer and I thought you'd like it." I did. It showed that he was intuitive, creative and that he cared.

The conversation that followed scared the crap

out of me. Without putting a clear label on exactly what was removed, or more importantly what remained in my head, we had gone from talking about a benign growth with others to a potentially deadly brain tumor.

Dr. Mahesh and his team seemed confident that there were strong options, and that highly qualified researchers and medical specialists were breaking new ground in cancer treatments every day. I have come to learn that that is true and while still a serious illness outcomes have dramatically improved.

However, there was still a real battle ahead. My apprehension was growing as new facts were presented. At one point, after the doctors left, I began softly sobbing. It was a total surprise and unstoppable. I remember a book by NBC News correspondent Betty Rollin, about her battle with breast cancer titled "First, You Cry." She is right. You have no choice.

In time, I felt better and looked forward to being released from neurosurgery and getting to work with the Summa oncologists.

I had become a fan.

6 - Heading Home

I had had enough of being in the hospital. It's so much easier to be lazy at home. I have made new connections and feel pretty good about the support systems that are forming. Monika and I made a friend a few years ago who was a resident on the staff at Summa and she had been through many of the treatments that I may be facing. She was there on that day and we had a good visit.

The next time you hear from me will be from Middleton Road in Hudson. As adventures go this will be protracted and dramatic, but I am convinced it will have *one of those endings that I love to write.*

Walking out of the hospital was a very uplifting experience. There was plenty of work left to be done and loads of questions, but while Monika was getting the car I had a chance to talk to Mr. Blevins, a double lung transplant recipient who had quite a story to tell. If you look around, it's not hard to find people with bigger challenges, problems and more dire circumstances than yours. Mr. Blevins was definitely one of those people, an old "street runner" who had made a mess of his life and he knew it. He had lost everything except his life and he still had plenty of bitterness.

Mr. Blevins was another study in contrast and I understood his entire ordeal. There was a point when he could only stay alive in a charity ward, his words, with IV lines in his fingers and dealing with shingles. He stretched out his hands and slowly moved fingers bowed at the knuckles in a vivid reenactment. It was easy to see in his jaundiced eyes that the memory echoed a whole new level of pain and discomfort. His wife on the other hand was dealing with her own fate and could not be there for him, he said. Implicit in his story was this poor woman, neglected and possibly abused watching the Old Street Man getting his due.

Mr. Blevins' outlook was limited, but in his tattered moments he, like many of us would, looked beyond the four walls of that vestibule to a Great Unknown and was totally convinced Something or Someone cared about him and had more work for him to do. He certainly did give me more hope, not that I didn't have plenty, but we can always use more.

There are so many tragic stories in an active and vital place such as Summa Akron City Hospital. There was a young man who was faced with such a virulent cancer that it seemed to be dismantling his formerly strong body right before our eyes. His girlfriend, also very young, was befuddled as she and her three year old son boarded the elevator after a very long stay. The little boy was curious about the staples in my head; on his face it was clear that his dominant emotion was fear.

We watch and read stories about these places, hospitals, detective squads, firehouses because the drama is constant. When it is so close we experience a different reaction, an intimacy that becomes real pain. Most of us want a dimmer switch for the pain.

But there is more that I have discovered: when it is happening to you the choices are stark, vivid and clear. Sadly the easiest choices seem to come from the embrace of anger and fear. I am convinced that they have the widest entry through the gateways to our emotions. It is always better to remain positive and confident in the knowledge that you will actually be better! Everyday there are indications some small, some large that this journey is leading to a better outcome.

Monika and I woke in the morning feeling grateful, she for having me home and me because she felt that way. We talked about our families and the good examples of family members meeting and beating challenges. Again, I am lucky because Mom and Dad, Al and Mary, were remarkable people. They learned tolerance and nimbleness in the age of Jim Crow laws and totally unreasonable restrictions on their ample talents and energy. The survivor instinct is a matter of degree, I am certain of it.

RoBBing Mind

The preceding pages were composed in the immediacy of a blog, as events unfolded. It was remarkable in its benefit to me as I was facing the <u>second</u> biggest challenge in my life.

The remainder is the book created with continuing information on my diagnosis, prognosis and reflections prompted by this new reality of living with —surviving — one of the most deadly forms of brain cancer.

7 - Fear

There is a basic concept by which many humans operate that a healthy fear is a life saving fear. And that is true. We don't put our hand in an open flame and we don't step off of a five-story balcony on the off chance that we actually can fly. But that same construct can also work against us.

As I was dealing with addiction more than two decades ago, the hardest battle was with the most nimble and ultimately invisible enemy: my own fears. When you pursue pleasure at all cost, without really doing anything to earn the elation, there are consequences. And they are never good, but add fear and they become the MOAF: The Mother Of All Fuckups. They hang on you like a bad smell, and you have physical reactions that are visible to almost anyone. These include things like sweating, darting eyes, loss of communication skills, loss of human sympathy or the ability to accurately read human signals. They become a bubble that surrounds you and prompts the question, "what's wrong with you?" I aways dreaded that question, yet I got it all the time.

Looking back I am reminded of those emotions and runaway feelings of utter doom, and I am reminded of that question, "what's wrong with you?" There is a vivid parallel between what happened to me then and what is happening now.

It does not have to be the result of disease. Certain conditions also bring about such inner turmoil that garners the same reaction. I've been told by some combat soldiers that there is a feeling when the smoke clears and the enemy is dead that they have earned more time, and have escaped fate. The feeling is not universal, but it is common.

Some people who have beaten the odds against serious illness also have that impression; that there was intervention or at least a measure of luck, training and maybe even good genes that kept that last moment from finding them where they stood.

Still, there remains the shadow of the tracer round, or the concussions that the guy next to them, the one who went through the same training, grew up in a similar town and was in that hellish place for primarily the same reason, yet was not so lucky. Those shadows can act as long knives in the night, preventing restful sleep and all the contributing issues of irritability and loss of focus and direction ("what's wrong with you?"). There might even be the distinct feeling that that bullet is still waiting, and if he or she remains in the combat zone, or in the early stages of a particular treatment protocol, those shadows will gain substance. Sadly we have plenty of combat vets returning who can better explain this unsettling feeling. It must have been a lot like this in the late 40's and 50's. We just wanted a period of calm, order and even predictability.

I am old enough to remember the pervasive fear blanketing our nation; that all could go up in a mushroom cloud at any second.

I was born as the Korean Conflict ended. They never called it a war back then. My father and mother never let fear stay in the house for very long. We watched TV all the time. The radio was a huge part of our mornings and our travels. But Mom and Dad always brought the focus back to us, back to being a family and doing what we had to do, even as the events of the world seemed so chaotic. They laughed easily and were generous, hard-working people.

As I calmed myself in middle of the night, dealing with this new crisis, I thought about all the possibilities and how (and why) I was not the other guy. Why was I not Howard, or the young man in his twenties who, as his pretty girlfriend said, "has more tumors than spine." With all respect to the courage of a warrior, it is not unlike looking at my buddy's lifeless, damaged body lying just steps away after the firefight. At least I am left with the same wonder.

And I will borrow their phrase: each day is a

bonus.

That notion is not distant nor vague; it hit home not that long ago. I have twin cousins with whom we spent a great deal of time during childhood. They were very special boys and men; supremely confident and comfortable in the knowledge that they were never really alone, never. By contrast I never had that connection. I was the youngest of three, but my brother, Al Jr. and sister, Barbara were adopted and though that was never an issue in our house – never mentioned – somehow I could feel it. My sister and brother looked a little different, but even that didn't matter we were very close. But it was not like having a twin, few things are. As we were growing into middle age (Lee and Lonnie were about 5 years my senior) we developed a real friendship as I did with many of my Kentucky cousins.

During the week when Lee, the slightly older brother, was to see his only daughter walk down the aisle, he suffered a fairly uncommon stroke. It was a basal artery thrombosis and it put a very strong guy on his back, down for the count. There was no return from this and both Lee and Lonnie knew it. Lee was a proud man and in spite of the blockage and subsequent damage he had time enough to say some things. I distinctly remember seeing him and hearing these words: "Polk, Chucky, I'm in trouble." The "Polk" was Willis Polk, the eldest son of

Grandmother's eldest boy, Ruben. "Chucky" was me, the only son born to Grandmother's first child. Willis was in training to be clergy and tried to take a role in Lee's funeral. Polk and Lee were best friends and he could not get through even half of what he wanted to say about the man. It had to be the most moving and profoundly painful funeral service I have ever attended. It hurts now just thinking about it.

Upon Lee's attack, Lonnie immediately got a medical checkup and found, to his shock, that he had the same potential for restrictive blood flow to this vital region of his brain. But there was a strange feature in the composition of these crucial arteries: Lonnie had developed a sort of bypass artery. It wasn't large, but it was there and mitigated the possibility of the same kind of massive stroke that took his brother, at least up until this point. Lonnie started paying attention to his blood pressure, what he ate and how he reacted to things. Already a calm person, he started accepting that he was very bright and deserving of the gifts of great kids, a beautiful wife and the respect of others.

Ruben and Mary Liza Polk had powerful and prolific offspring. And I love and respect all my cousins, but in my view Grandmother's baby girl, Ann and her rock-solid husband Robert Jackson Jr., seemed to produce the strongest limbs in that family tree: Lee, Lonnie, Linda and Leslie. I am very proud to call them family, along with the Polks, the Bibbs and Parkers.

I spoke to Lonnie shortly after my initial diagnosis and have since the surgery. He and I have adopted a brotherly connection for one another. It is defiantly one of the perks of surviving this challenge.

As I write this (Sunday, July 28, 2013) news came across that a long-time Dallas/National morning radio host Kidd Kraddick passed away yesterday near New Orleans. Kraddick was an inspiration in that he could balance humor, edgy nuance and still be safe to listen to with kids in the car. That took a great deal of skill and hard work. But he loved it and he was very much admired. I bring this up now, in this particular section because Kidd was 53 years old and a sudden death like that is almost always cardiovascular or neurologically related.

Was that the bullet intended for me? There are so many things that have revealed themselves forcing me to quiet down and watch the road markers. Something more important than we ever thought possible is on my horizon and I tend to think, if you look for it, on yours, too.

9 - A Moment With God

Many of you reading this are on a scale that ranges
from devout believers in a specific, historical notion of
God, faith and religion, to a convention that such
thoughts are superstitions and manifestations of an
uninformed if not a weak intellect. There are those
who have explored the teaching of ancient cultures
and how they apply thought, deed and intentions into
a better way to live.

I have often said that the only difference
between me in September 1986, a drug addicted drunk,
and me today is that on October first of that year I
learned a simple prayer. That prayer has since
expanded, but it started out this way: before I step too
far from my bed I get on my knees and say, "God,
please keep me sober today." At night, before climbing
into bed I repeat the process and say, "God, thank
You for keeping me sober today." So far, for nearly 26
years, it has worked.

Of course there were other things to do, but
the notion that I had turned-in my simple request to a
power I have no hope of ever understanding made the
difference. Some might interpret that as calling on my
own sense of strength and determination to avoid

drinking or using drugs. But why were those abilities so dormant before I started praying?

In my opinion my friends devoted strictly to science are not entirely wrong, and my religious friends are not entirely correct. The reason this worked then and still does is because part of my addicted personality is a massive ego! When I spend those twice daily moments with God, I am asking a universal power, whatever that might be, to pay attention to *me!* Take a little of that magic and give this guy a break, just for today. We'll deal with tomorrow tomorrow. In those moments of humility and faith I feel emboldened to trust that something has my back and I can do what I need to do without worrying about feeding my ego with intoxicants.

Lots of drunks feel superior because they buy into the illusion brought about by the drink or drugs. But I have learned that mist is mist and eventually it all falls to the floor as dirty water. If I really want to confirm my specialness, my exceptionalism I must perform as I profess, I must *walk the walk.*

In the beginning I tested this notion often. My career was in shambles, my family, except for Mary Collins, was non-existent, and all I really had was an ability to orate glibly. In AA meetings the lack of inhibition and vocation that involved public speaking was both useful and a distraction. Yet as the veil began to dissolve I noticed that people were looking at me differently, there was a spark of honest appreciation, if not admiration. Moving away from the false stage erected by booze and cocaine the real actor began showing up, and he wasn't terrible. In fact he was getting better! That was far more useful and exciting than any drug.

Today I have a God of my understanding, and perhaps more importantly One who understands me. And yes, I believe that relationship is Supernatural. So for those who ask, "where is the proof?" In simple terms there is no proof other than my personal experience and just like the autumn of 1986, this summer of 2013, has reinforced what I am about to say: there is far greater proof of a power guiding the universe down to the smallest detail than there is that it is all randomly (or even structurally) colliding principles of physics. You see, I think too much of me for that kind of happenstance and I definitely think too much of you.

In the case of brain tumors and potentially brain cancer, where does this foundation come in? It guides me out of the woods. It restores my faith that though lightening can and does strike twice, in the words of my dear friend Terry Gordon, "no storm lasts forever."

10 - Little Big Books

What began as a therapeutic cure for waiting and not knowing has transformed into a roadmap for hope in a small book. I am reminded of another small book that had a profound impact on me: Dr. Viktor Frankl's *Man's Search for Meaning.* In a diminutive 168 page memoir, Dr. Frankl takes readers into the depths of hopelessness and inhumanity – Nazi death camps — to find perhaps and greatest humanity of all. If you are not familiar with it I highly recommend the brief, albeit powerful read.

I was exposed to this book at an early age by an unusual mentor, a graduate student in mathematics who was a fraternity brother with my dad. They were Alphas, one of the earliest of the academic fraternities among black men in America. Most were educators and scientists, preachers and medical doctors. It was an answer to the then restricted Phi Beta Kappa society.

Alfred Armstead was the son of an Alabama share cropper who was born with an off-the-chart IQ and an intense curiosity. He was eccentric in the extreme and would have frightened most parents to have him around their impressionable 8 year old. But Mary Collins took a different view. She trusted Alfred to do no harm and that he would actually open my world. She was right. He would usually come by on Saturdays when mom and dad were out to one of their many, often formal functions. We would do homework and play chess. He would talk about mathematical theories and actually make them fun, fun for a 3rd grader!

Alfred made the determination early that I was not the mathematical type, but I excelled in the human sciences of history, philosophy and literature. He took me to the Great Lakes Shakespeare Festival that was thriving in our city at the time and helped me understand the meanings, historical context and even the language of the great playwright. He guided me to the real world of abstracts. He knew there were plenty of living and breathing monsters to hold this boy's interests.

But there were times when his extreme methods were, on the surface, confusing. One of the things he did was re-purpose Nazi Germany! Alfred would often dress, smoke and talk as a Gestapo operative (black trench coat, fedora and remarkable accent.) It was great fun for me. It worked toward building our little community and an imaginative vehicle for some hard lesions about life and perceptions. Alfred would never let the pretext of the most horrific time and system of government the world has known go unchallenged. What he did was fill the stage, ask the question and give an impressionable young mind the freedom to explore the possibilities. How could the German State, built first on pride and determination devolve into a society of murder and hubris that threatened the entire world? Alfred showed me how. It was risky and, honestly, brilliant. The child grew into a man who had a willingness to apply more than just the notion of evil to human events. You will see that this education has helped me over the years and in an odd way prepared me for what awaits.

11- Look for the Best…

…Expect the worst and take what God sends you. This is a sentence anyone from Mary Liza's bloodline can complete unaided. It was Grandmother's credo and although it is not entirely original it resonated through some radically difficult times.

Ours, like many southern black families – then and now – was a matriarch. Black men tended to fall into one of two categories: skilled or unskilled. Some fought the system of bigotry and oppression from within battling demons that often amounted to alcoholism, crime or the complex misogyny similar to that dramatized by George Gershwin in *Porgy and Bess*. Life in the time of my grandparents was not without simple pleasures. But it was hard. They lived on a gravel lane that was bounded by small shares of subsistence gardens, a large tobacco field and terminated in a small stream called a "branch." Across the field and stream were moderately large houses with big back yards and white children playing happily.

In spite of all this, the Polks were the lucky ones. My grandfather was skilled. He knew how to use a tool box and he was strong, smart and sober enough to stay employed even during the toughest times.

Ruben Polk loved to work and he loved his wife and kids. A quiet man with a sweet smile and arms that could snap a pine, few people challenged him. His father-in-law was a minister in a small church in nearby town called Midway. That job held much more power than just preaching to the faithful. For that reason, Rev. Willis Garnett sent two of his sons to school. One became a doctor in Chicago; the other a talented and coveted house manager – a valet - in New York City.

Having married Rev's oldest and prettiest daughter, Reuben was not about the let the minister down. He and his wife – who cleaned houses until well into her seventies and was as charming and talented as any women I have ever known - had a plan to make sure their children were educated and made it out of that Tobacco Row.

Mary Liza had two boys and four girls. It was the girls who guided the family, led by Mary Bohannon, my mother. She excelled beyond the limits of that small town and was sent to Evanston near Chicago to live with her uncle Dr. John Garnett and receive a city high school education before going on to a teacher's college back in Frankfort, Kentucky.

It's important to note that although the plight of descendents of slaves in most of the country was blighted and desperate, Kentucky maintained an ambiguity before, during the Civil War and continued throughout the seemingly endless stretch of time when

Jim Crow laws sought to maintain a clearly dominant white American culture throughout the nation.

While I wished the men in Mary Liza's clan were as strong as their father, sadly Reuben died too soon to completely imprint upon them the true nature of being a man. This was a young boy's observation and my cousins might disagree.

Both Reuben and Wayman had challenges, mostly with alcoholism and a general frustration. But they both worked, perhaps never missing a day on the job. And they married women who fit the Polk mold very well, especially Reuben's wife Margaret who stayed by Mary Liza's side for the remainder of the Grand lady's life.

And the men whom the sisters married provided moral leadership and they did well. As mentioned, the limbs of the Polk tree are very strong, filled with Jacksons, Parkers, Polks, Collinses and Bibbs, many of whom have made a real difference.

Now the only one remaining is Ann, the youngest. She is the mother of the twins, Lee and Lonnie part of whose story you have read. Ann also had a daughter and another son.

Before we leave the Bluegrass I need to share a picture of Grandmother that is in my head. She is standing at the top of Macy Ave., the town of Versailles, 50's era cars and a gentle street blurred and gray in the distance. My grandmother has a wide-brimmed hat on, I believe it is straw with a narrow veil just over her eyes, a dark fitted suit and the slightest smile highlighted by the sun. Her head is tilted to the right and her chin was held high. That moment in time spoke to me all my life. It was reassuring and even when she passed away the long reach of that powerful woman pulled me from many difficulties. I can see it now and I know she is doing it again.

12 - The Hidden Hand

William Styron, a brave and insightful writer, was diagnosed with severe depression later in his life. Of course he wrote about it. The book is called *Darkness Visible*. In it he wrote about the silent invasion of mental illness. I cannot approach the level of his understanding as to what was happening to him, except to recommend the work.

Depression has always been a concern of mine. Although never diagnosed with the condition, I know what it feels like and remain on my guard that it does not leach into this experience. A positive attitude is fragile especially when facts and possibilities seem to generate more conflict than harmony.

There is a key to avoiding that darkness and that is facing it head-on, similar to steering into the slide on an icy road. If you've tried it you know it is not an easy thing to do but it works and next time you are prepared.

Another book I have been exposed to on this journey is Jill Bolte Taylor's *My Stroke of Insight*. It is a wildly popular story of a Harvard trained neuroanatomist who suffered a stroke in exactly the wrong place in her brain. Dr. Bolte Taylor has struggled throughout the last 15 years to retrain her thinking and return, not only to a productive life, but to a new world in which she can share her struggles. Dr. Bolte Taylor is on a remarkable path that, unlike my case, started in negative territory. The difference is that her formal training allowed her to track the progress of her disease almost from the beginning.

I highly recommend the book and the multimedia presentations Dr. Bolte Taylor has produced.

Among these gifted people there is a moment when all the talent, fame and relative success in the world cannot prevent epic calamity. It might be a course correction similar to what has happened to me, or a heart-breaking reality such as the horrific accident that happened to the only son of my friend Terry Gordon. Tyler Gordon is alive, but his struggles are profound. And while we can reconcile so many things as they happen to us, we don't always see what is going on inside those we love. In many respects, whether loved one or caregiver, the true impact seems to remain a great mystery. I see that in Monika, Terry and others. They care so much and give so much that they often don't recognize the drain on their own well-being.

My friend Joe McGee, the news videographer and reporter who presented my return to the WAKR airwaves for Cleveland's NewsNet 5, has a son who suffered tremendous brain damage during a motorcycle accident several years ago. Joe tells me that his son is about 80% back and happily working at a nearby restaurant. Joe's exact words were, "he is grateful."

The good news is much of what happens is dictated by our attitude and our attitude is fueled by our gratitude. It may seem simplistic. But I have found they are inextricably linked.

You will see (and have seen) many times throughout this work that I am sure a positive attitude has saved me from the worst of it. That attitude starts by taking an honest inventory of the things I have, the gains made and even the bullets missed, for whatever reason, and being thankful for each one.

With that in mind, one of my neurosurgeons characterized this tumor as the "guilt free cancer," because there was nothing done, or not done as far as the research shows, to cause the tumor to appear. It is an interesting way to think of something so dangerous and demanding.

Grateful beats guilty any day.

13 - Spiders, Ol' Mr. P and the Fear Hammer

"It is clear that all of our problems, personal and universal stem from the over-supply of, and undue power given to fear." ~AA Sponsor Ron W.

Most of us have some healthy and some irrational fears. Fear helps us avoid serious harm, but when fear rules your life it can be as debilitating as, well, a brain tumor.

As a child I was frightened to death by spiders, to the point that I would wake up in the night and violently shake out my sheets and pillowcases until I was sure that no 8-legged visitor had invaded my bed. This continued as we camped across the country in 1961 and engaged in all kinds of outdoor activities as I was growing up.

I once told Alfred of my fears and how there was nothing he could say, as smart as he was that could change the way I felt. Alfred, tilted his head a bit to the right and said, "More people are injured on slick sidewalks than ever by *Latrodectus*." It was the first time that I ever heard the genus name for the source of my horror, but it intrigued me. Were we talking about the same thing?

That evening we set off to discover the true nature of the little beasts. We attacked it in much the same way that we had researched other topics, except that I shivered any time we turned a page that potentially had a color plate with images of long spindly legs, multiple eyes or worse, a close up of streaked, black inverted fangs.

After a while the bugs became as innocuous as Lewis and Clark, ancient Egypt, or the unconventional approach we had taken in the study of the Third Reich. Slowly the subject no longer was fearsome, but a thing to be studied. Alfred and I had hammered that fear into a topic, and topics don't terrorize.

I even used the work to earn an "A" in a science class in which I was struggling.

Suddenly I learned that by exploring something I enjoyed in a paper, I could atone for all the wasted time during the school year. It worked all the way through high school, and in some respects I am doing the same thing now.

As Mary Collins entered her mid 70's, her beautiful, top of the black board hand writing became halting and inconsistent. She knew something was not quite right. It was getting difficult for her to get out of bed in the morning and as a new widow she found all the things that my dad had done for her hard to replicate.

Mom was substitute teaching to supplement her retirement income and she loved the elementary school kids, but her physical failings were getting in the way. She also still loved thoroughbred racing and she was a great handicapper, but sitting in the grand stands was not as comfortable as it once had been.

Parkinson's disease was in headlines then, primarily because of President Ronald Reagan's shaking hands and halting diction. Mary Collins refused to acknowledge that she might have succumbed to the same vitality-robbing nerve disorder as the President. If I mentioned Parkinson's, she would correct me by saying, "it's just o'l Mr. P, grabbing my hand for a minute."

I thought I would try and help her come to terms with her fears by applying the same technique I used to defuse my fear of spiders. I researched Parkinson's disease and would catch Mom in moments when she would just want to hear my voice and then drop a few tid-bits about the disorder. She would listen patiently and wait until there was a fact that she could dispute, thereby proving, at least to her satisfaction, that she simply was not a candidate for Parkinson's

Ultimately Ol' Mr. P took a back seat to late onset diabetes and hydrocephalus, which required delicate neurosurgery to give her another five years of reasonably comfortable life. What I learned from Mary Collins during this time is what I call *the dignity of decline*.

Mary Collins would not complain and never blamed her situation on anyone or anything. That is not to say that she didn't have needs, notably the need to relieve the profound loneliness endemic in elder care. That was up to us, Monika and me. I wish I could say I was a champion here, much like she was my champion through almost all of my life. There were days when I came late to visit her and left much too soon. Most days I was there, helping her with lunch and getting her cleaned up and then sitting in the sun. But Mrs. Collins, as I sometimes called her in honor of her life-long devotion to teaching, remained true to her nature to the very end.

When that day came, she and I listened to Lena Horn singing Stormy Weather. I sang along with one of the 20th Century's biggest African-American stars, and a woman to whom mom was often compared.

That late afternoon, with hospice staff in the background, her breathing became horse and slowed. My heart sunk, knowing that I was about to say goodbye for the last time.

The proud woman worked to keep her face calm, as though she knew — even with eyes closed — how much pain I was in. Then she frowned a bit. I can only imagine that she realized that there was nothing more to do.

Then in a moment of profound courage she became peaceful, sent one more breath from her lungs, and remained quiet. Mary Collins finally left her baby boy there at her bedside, giving him permission to press on.

No fear, ever.

One note: Not long after Mary Collins departed, Alfred also passed away. The difference was remarkable. Alfred Armstead was robbed of his mind by dementia and Alzheimer's. I spoke to him on the telephone in the last days of his life, unable to go to Colorado to see him. He was frightened and the man who saw things few could see, understood things few could hope to comprehend, was drowning in confusion and a sense of abandonment. Death was likely a welcome relief.

14- Inelegant Exits

Sprinkled throughout this book are stories of brave men and woman facing seemingly insurmountable challenges with dignity and determination. Sadly that is not necessarily the rule. It might even be the exception.

Here are some examples of losing the battle before beginning the fight.

In mid August I attended the grave-side burial of an old friend. I had not seen him in many years and his condition was unknown to me. It turns out he had had heart surgery about ten years prior and things did not go well. It happens more often than we might want to know. My friend Jay was an accomplished engineer/artist in a very challenging field. It was a sedentary job before the introduction of computers and when that world became dominated by digital tools it only got worse for him.

Jay used to jog a few miles daily and was generally health conscious. At some point all that changed. He started gaining weight so that by the time his heart problems came about he was morbidly obese. At the time of his death his 5 foot 6 inch frame was incapable of carrying the 450 pounds he had amassed. Jay was my age and he had given up.

Unless we are in the skin of another we cannot fully appreciate the difficulty of facing the challenge of fighting a life-threatening disease compounded by threats posed by our own demons. Jay is the second example of this kind of surrender in the year 2013. The other example had fought a congenital disease that required hours of painful daily treatments. One day we got a call from his wife, he, too, was ready to surrender. The fight had reached its limit.

While these relatively young men were handed difficult fates, the challenge of obesity was overpowering for both of them just as it is for many others. Losing 100 pounds or more under good conditions is daunting, trying to do so with heart-lung issues or other organ failure could be viewed as justifiably impossible.

But the third example is so horrifying that I must issue a warning here. Not only is this exit unkind, but it is an example of such extreme disease of the mind, body and soul as to render it the stuff of fiction. Yet like everything else in this book it is totally true.

Tibor was my Monika's father and he was a man who defied logic and basic human instincts. Were you to have met him, you might have thought he was just a nice older man with a thick accent and a clumsy, if not charming naïveté. Only the thick accent would be accurate.

Tibor truly believed he was the smartest man on the planet. He would collect newspapers just to pit one article against another to prove Popes, presidents, scientists and Nobel laureates were morons. His points were flimsy at best, but in his mind there was ironclad proof that every person in authority was completely incompetent.

This was harmless except that his only joy was hurting those who were closest to him. Tibor also believed that rules did not apply to him, no rules. He would eat cheese pizza that was months, if not years old. He would go weeks without showering and once, when his wife was on an extended stay in Europe, he slept on the same sheets for 6 months without washing them (or himself). Aside from the smell, his house remained orderly with odd technology supporting his self-perceived creativity.

One of Tibor's favorite targets was his stepson, a very bright, shy young man who was devoted to his family. For his commitment the only reward was ridicule and humiliation from his stepfather. It would often break my heart to see this in action and I would stick up for the young man. In a string of racist insults spoken in Hungarian — which Tibor believed I could not possibly understand — he would dismiss my aid and continue the verbal abuse.

At one point Tibor got sick. Rather than do the small things to get better, it was time to show the doctors that he was the superior being.

My farther-in-law developed a sty in his left eye. Simple enough to fix, but his insanity turned a tiny infection into a slide toward one of the most brutal ends imaginable.

Tibor's proclamation was this, "you are doctor, you went to university for years, you fix me." The only problem is Tibor refused to do the smallest things the doctors recommended except take medication, mostly antibiotics and only then when he felt like it. When told to put warm compresses on the area he would put the compress on his other eye, or his foot, never in the affected place. He would even do things so vile as to render the compress not only non therapeutic, but unsanitary.

Discomfort prompted him to pick at the location with dirty tweezers or industrial tools, only to show up at an appointment accusing the doctors of making matters worse. Matters got worse, much worse.

The infection, left basically untreated by an uncooperative patient, began to spread and gain in strength and speed. It invaded his cheek and sinuses eventually killing tissue until the entire left side of his face began to peel away. The malignancy eventually entered the vital glands in his head and neck and in less than a year Tibor was doomed.

Almost to the end, as his sardonic grin of exposed teeth, gum, temporal muscles and jaw bones, made his appearance worthy of the finest horror make-up artist. Still he remained defiant. "This is what your medicine and education did to me!" He spat.

When Tibor died, his wife, ever devoted in spite of the nightmares he invented for her, was by his side. And so was the one daughter whom he often found the most pleasure in hurting, my Monika. His last moments were painful and grotesque.

It occurred to me in those last hours that Tibor finally got his wish; to be proven correct and that this life was an ugly sham. It certainly was the case for him, and he died with the hurt and shame he tried to heap on others right there on his tattered face.

Peace came to his wife and she is happy now with a man who is her best friend. My Monika still lets echoes of her father's abuse seep in and harm her all over again. But she also has a best friend who will spend a lifetime defending her from those demons. That, of course is her husband for whom she is caring now in heroic fashion and always with love and devotion. And it is returned in kind.

My father in law was always a curiosity to me, truly foreign in so many ways, capable of compassion toward strangers for no apparent reason yet so hateful and mean to those closest to him. Clearly Monika retained none of his DNA, at least nothing related to personality and demeanor.

15 -The World's Oldest DJ

My business and craft has been radio for as long as I can remember. I built a small crystal radio at age 7, but more than that I studied Radio in America. What I discovered was a unique marriage of science, necessity and marketing. Once a matter of national security, it quickly occupied an important place in the nation's living rooms. In times of war and peace, change and stagnation, the first mass media was a wide canvass capable of many forms.

Music was a natural for the radio and it performed live from some of the most famous ballrooms in the country. But the thing that made radio a national obsession was and is the spoken word, be it deadly serious tones of FDR telling the nation that war was unavoidable following the attack on Pearl Harbor, or the news of quickly shifting events as witnessed and reported by Edward R. Murrow and others. It was also human dramas, real or fictional. Situation comedies, melodramas, mysteries and varieties filled the broad airwaves several nights a week.

Through it all a new art form was being created and a new term was formed in broadcast facilities around the world: radio voice. It meant a deep, clear instrument trained to enunciate the most complicated words. These men — and they were almost all men — developed an interesting erudition when it came to the spoken word, not quite American in dialect and not quite continental, but somewhere between everyone's farther and the ultimate authority.

As public figures began using the media it was clear that a new set of skills was needed and a new understanding of communicating not only to those in attendance, but also to the unseen millions listening to their radios.

While Franklin Roosevelt was a master of this art, his Uncle, Teddy, with his thin tenor voice was a marked failure. When Woodrow Wilson suffered a stroke later in his term the affected voice of the President did little to instill confidence. FDR could broadcast from a chair and no one would think to question his abilities either physically or as the leader of a nation. But a President with dysarthria — that distinctive disability of speech often associated with stroke victims — has little hope of sending a positive message.

As important as politics were in the first half of the 20th Century, it was entertainment that guided the medium post war and today. Add to that medium the visuals of television and the electronic media captured the culture unabated.

Perhaps the most famous Radio and TV personality who evolved solely from the sheer power of youth and music was Dick Clark. His pleasing demeanor and genuine love for the music and the kids was just what a war weary culture needed. Clark helped in no small way to defuse racial tensions through music and entertainment, and while Walter Cronkite narrated our launch into a modern age, Dick Clark and others like him provided the sound track, as free and forward flying as any Apollo rocket.

In December of 2004, just weeks away from the iconic TV show *Dick Clark's Rockin' New Year's Eve*, the voice of youth suddenly turned into the voice of age and infirmity by what was believed to be a mild stroke. While he fared pretty well for a man in his mid seventies with multiple health issues, the affect of dysarthria was all the listener heard. And while the love for Dick Clark never faded, his skills as a broadcaster were in rapid decline.

Dick Clark and his heir apparent Ryan Seacrest made the last New Year's Rockin' Eve by rockin' and ringin' in 2012. There was something heroic about the appearance. Dick Clark died in April of that year. But in many ways his life was over when stroke robbed him of his voice.

I am by no means comparing myself and my local radio career to the great Dick Clark, but the fear of my voice being robbed by this brain tumor and subsequent treatments begs the comparison. Were dysarthria to compress and distort my speech my career would be over.

As you will see, distorted speech might be the least of my worries.

16 – Love Fest

I was back at WAKR for a visit just two weeks from my initial surgery. My friend and colleague Ed Esposito arranged for a TV-digital news person to come in and record a segment with me for NewsNet 5. It was profoundly moving.

There are things that happen to friends that give you two distinctly different reactions. The first is, "thank God it wasn't me." The second is, "Man! I'm glad that he's okay." These are both genuine and pretty common. I realized that the people at Rubber City Radio Group are really my family in more ways than I realized before this crisis and for that I am truly grateful.

Modern medicine has made my story less unique. That is the story as I understood it on that beautiful Tuesday morning and for that reason I wanted to keep things in perspective. When I tell you that I was in danger, I can attribute much of that to apprehension. Looking back a number of days later, and understanding the real struggles faced by those with profound brain trauma and disability, I wanted to remain circumspect, at least that was my reality and the one that was recorded and still exists on line.

I still did not know the total story, the confirmation I was to get in just a few days. Brain tumors were serious, but there was as good a chance that it was benign as anything else. I projected good health and a good pace of recovery. It would have been the case no matter what the news that awaited. I was determined to start the process from a positive and winning attitude regardless.

That determination was about to be put to the test.

I sold my gun today
Aside from the fact that we need the money, I didn't feel comfortable with a firearm in the house. This goes along with what I am learning about the unpredictability of the human brain. That is not to say that I believe I would suddenly lose touch with reality and harm my family or anyone. It is to say we can never be completely sure.

17 – The Verdict

August 1, 2013

A big news day in Northeast Ohio; an especially horrifying kidnapping trial has finally ended with a plea deal for Ariel Castro. This mousey little man had confined three young women, fathered a child with one and for ten years held these girls, now young women in his dilapidated home on Cleveland's west side. It was a story that captured the attention and in many ways the hearts and anger of a nation.

The drama was intensified by the fact that, in spite of the awful decade of abuse, they did survive even as some friends, neighbors even family had thought they were lost forever. Castro was on live local and national news, seeming to justify his despicable actions.

His former captives have become celebrities of sorts, if reluctantly. But Cleveland is the kind of place that holds onto good news, because there has been so much bad news over the years. This story set up a summer that still has had plenty of horror, but with the rescue of Gina, Michelle and Amanda in the headlines, it seemed a little warmer, a little sunnier.

This was also the day I got the definitive results from the pathology examination of my brain tumor.

The news was to be delivered by Dr. Paul H., the neurosurgeon who extracted as much of the mass as could be safely removed. Monika and I were ready for the worst; we had agreed on that long before. But when the doctor came into the examination room, before any meaningful information was exchanged, we knew that this was not good news.

He quickly and almost painlessly took the staples from my scalp and sat down, opened a folder and waited, as though I could tell him what was in this manila binder, I could have.

My tumor is a glioblastoma multiforme or GBM, fourth level - advanced. Dr. H. was gentle, but straight forward. It is the type of tumor that tends to return and even move about the brain (grow and go), if and when it does it will make a real mess of things. Monika and I sat and digested these facts. At one point she wanted to say something and I did the rudest thing, I held up my hand effectively quieting her, I'm not sure if I wanted Dr. H. to complete his thought or if I wanted to say something I thought profound. Regardless, it was exactly the wrong thing to have done. Monika is in this as much as I am, perhaps even more emotionally invested. She is the one, should the time come, to deal with the outward consequences of a malignant brain tumor not only robbing my mind but stealing *her* life as well as mine. She is the one who sat by my bedside and prayed over me, cried over me and worried herself sick. I promised her I would never do that again.

Still there was more good news than bad. The location of the tumor and the surgical site was pretty good for me. It was located in a spot where I can continue to stay who I am, at least for the time being. And even if it grows again this type of cancer tends to stay isolated in the right brain and affect left side functions, the most destructive being my speech. It is still unpredictable and a new tumor can show up almost any place in the brain including very dangerous locations such as the brain stem causing rapid decline.

Were this 10 years ago – 5 years ago - doctors would have been far less optimistic about this diagnosis. They would have offered treatments but very little hope. In many respects it is good to have this part, the wondering and projecting out of the way. We know what it is and we are just beginning to understand how to fight it.

But there is much more to this part of the process — the surgical options — and while we were fortunate to have a talented neurosurgeon perform with remarkable skills and positive results, in many respects we were just entering the starting gate.

18 – Labels

This is not the first time that I have been diagnosed with a potentially fatal disease, although most people would not place alcoholism in the same category as brain cancer.

Twenty six years ago my life was over, at least that is the way it seemed. Mornings brought regret, nights brought chaos and the days were a precarious balance on a knife edge. That is the life of a drug addict and alcoholic. That was my life and it was draining into oblivion faster than imaginable.

Put into perspective, of those with this type of cancer there is about a 35% survival rate although that statistic is skewed by many factors. If you compare these facts: fewer than 10,000 people are diagnosed with GBM per year and fewer still with a grade 4 tumor, while those with my level of addiction and use in the mid-80's also had a less than 50% survival rate then the similarities become clear. If you factor in alcohol related automobile fatalities and suicide the numbers rise dramatically. Taken in context then you might agree that the two conditions share bleak outcomes.

In the case of GBM traditional and advanced treatments have lengthened the time before possible recurrence. Other factors seem to aid in positive outcomes.

I've attempted here to give you some insight as to how to stay upbeat and trust that beginning with a positive attitude and maintaining a positive outlook can make a tremendous difference. But there is really no proof that how I feel about this condition has anything to do with my prognosis, just as many people will tell me that inner strength and determination changed me from being a drunk to a non-drinking productive adult. I can't prove them wrong or right and there are other books and media on that topic.

Here is where I can make a strong argument that there is more than science in human survival and I will use that same topic, one that I know well.

Before 1900 the accepted scourge of the nation and the world was alcoholism. In a cry heard in churches and social organization drunkenness was deemed the destroyer of the family and thereby halting the progress of a new nation. Even now substance abuse can account for an astonishing number of deaths in America; by some estimates more than 75,000 when you include suicide and traffic fatalities.

By 1930 the country had tried and failed prohibiting all use of alcohol and soon discovered two things: The government can only dictate so much when it comes to human behavior and where there is a vacuum in human desire there are enterprising criminals who will rush in to fill it.

But something else that happened around the time of Prohibition's repeal is good people decided to learn more about alcoholism and tackle the problem using a different approach. Many pioneers in the treatment of alcoholism were associated with the hospital that played a vital role in my recovery from brain cancer. St. Thomas Hospital in Akron, now a part of the Summa Health Care System, is credited with facilitating the first meeting between the founders of Alcoholics Anonymous, consistently recognized as having long-term success with helping men and women get and stay sober. But even with that over 70 year track record, success is still a 50-50 proposition.

As I have described the cascading events that led to a plan for treating brain cancer, my introduction to addiction recovery was also a process. It began more than 10 years before the day I walked into my first AA meeting.

In 1976 my only brother, Al Jr., was faced with what he thought was a terrible reality. He was sexually ambiguous. He loved dressing up as a woman, but he also loved women and I never got any indication that he was homosexual. Believing he might be gay probably scared him more than did his unusual urges. It was a confusing and painful thing for our father to comprehend.

Al was never much of a drinker or drug user, not like I was. As hard as he fought against his personal conflicts his dangerous slide did not occur until intoxicants entered his troubled world.

It was as though he was given permission to finally end the confusion and pain that he must have felt every day of his short life. The only answer, his only solution to this darkness was on the crumbling ledge of a high bridge in the middle of Cleveland, Ohio.

My brother had made two attempts to end his life. The second try he succeeded. His body hit the filthy Cuyahoga River at near terminal velocity and amid the heavy marine oil and other pollutants almost every bone shattered upon impact before he slowly sank into the mire.

As one of the Cleveland Police river patrol officers who helped pull my brother's body from the Cuyahoga put it, "it's like hitting an unbreakable glass wall, or a block of ice. There's just no give at all."

My father and I drove to Cleveland's morgue to identify my brother. I could not do it, and I will never forget my dad's expression when he left that viewing room. It might have been the most pain I have ever seen on that strong face, a face that looked then a lot like mine does now.

Ten years later my father passed away. It happened suddenly on one Tuesday morning in July. He was my hero in so many ways and when he left I, too was lost. Two months later I had had enough. And

I believe God listened to my call for help. I tried to fight addiction on my own but that was not working.

October 1, 1986 was a Wednesday night. It was raining. I was wearing a windbreaker from Grumman Aviation, the last place my brother had worked with dignity. The three mile walk was lonely, but something was carrying me along, or so it seemed, and I was out of options. Behind me was an empty second floor suite. The apartment was filthy; the kitchen reeked with a new level of foul smells and the bed hadn't been slept in for months.

Monika had moved out almost a year before. But she had left a pair of shoes in our tiny closet. I don't know why. Seeing those shoes, small and delicate, always made me cry.

By the time I made it to the large, classically designed Catholic Church, I was soaked and felt like a drowned rat. At the door was Ralph. He looked to me like a real-life incarnation of an R. Crumb comic character; badly in need of a haircut and a wardrobe update. But he held out his hand, took mine in a strong handshake and said, "Welcome. You're in the right place."

It was the first of many greetings at AA meetings. By the time that meeting was over I felt right at home.

For the first six months I introduced myself this way: "I'm an alcoholic and my name is Chuck." I led with this label for years. When among other alcoholics I put that part of me right up front.

Now there is another label, another community to which I belong, not by habit or propensity but by disease, a biological fact and how it will end is still a moving target.

I am certain that I will be a brain tumor/brain cancer survivor, but unlike the useful knowledge that even after two and a half decades I am still an alcoholic and still recovering day by day. I'm not sure that constant reminder would be as therapeutic regarding brain cancer.

19 - From 12 You Get 3

The foundation for Alcoholics Anonymous is articulated in Twelve Steps. It is nothing new, you can find the number 12 in man's most ancient attempts at organizing life, the universe and everything. From the planets of the Zodiac to the Disciples of Christ and lesser known groupings, man has embraced the dozen.

When the structure of this new type of approach to getting and staying sober was born, so were twelve distinct, suggested instructions that could be duplicated regardless of the individual or the extent with which addiction had taken hold.

Rather than going over the steps – they can easily be found should you need them – I will break it down to a basic three: Trust that the Universe (God of your understanding) is bigger than you; dump your guilt; help others who are in the same mess. It's really that simple and I believe it can apply to anything. We seem to be wired to the understanding that there are greater things in this world, if not beyond, than our own petty worries and fears. Even the strict scientist has an almost unnatural adherence to the laws of science, so much so that when innovation or discovery shakes their understanding there is an almost visceral reaction.

Another concept that seems hard wired in our nature is guilt. We steep in it and the worst part about guilt is that it knows no end. We can feel guilty about something we did a decade ago or tomorrow, it doesn't matter and unless we make a concerted effort to eradicate it the negative impact will return again and again. Guilt and feeling guilty is about as useless as worry, yet we engage both far too much and far too often.

Dumping guilt is a process according to the 12 step program and it begins by forgiving oneself then setting out to seek, if not the forgiveness, at least the acknowledgement of contrition from those we might have hurt. It's not easy, but I found it to be the most freeing of the processes.

Helping others struggling with addiction, in the case of staying sober, means sharing experiences that might be helpful. It also means listening, really listening from a place of understanding. This also gets us out of our own problems. This is the enduring practice that has allowed AA to grow and remain successful.

The beauty of AA is also that nobody got rich off it, not the founders, not the leaders today, mainly because there are no leaders. It is truly a collective organism that grows larger and lighter with every new member stumbling in from the rain to be greeted by a sincere handshake.

I don't know what Glioblastoma Multiforme will do to me. It will not be as easy to treat as simply not taking a drink today. But somehow I think that even using just 3 of 12 pieces of sound advice can tip the scales in my favor.

Faith and History

I wish I could say that Monika shares my optimism. She can, but not without some help.

In our more than 35 years together we have had more challenges than successes. We (to be fair, I) have run through at least two fortunes and had life and death dramas that did not defeat us.

As I was falling into the last stages of addiction in 1985 we divorced. Monika was able to pick up her life where she left off with her sister and mother and a wonderful 4 year old child, Poppy. This little girl was co-parented by the three women, her mother Cecilia, grandmother Omi and Aunt Monika. My role was important in her life but still compromised by alcoholism and distrust.

Monika never gave up on me and looking back, although my disease and behavior prevented us from staying together, the love we had for one another never waned.

When I entered recovery that love blossomed and in two years we were remarried. We remained devoted to that family and it was strengthened at least for Poppy and Omi. Cecilia still had battles to wage and today she is doing fine. Poppy is a remarkable young professional who has a drive for public service. Omi left us in the spring of 2012 and her last years were as loving and comfortable as an 87 year old could hope for thanks to Monika.

I think it is important to recall these events because at any given time they could have appeared hopeless and all we had was faith that things will turn out for the best.

My friend Tony often says 'wishful thinking is no strategy.' He is correct, but faith and history are powerful reminders that believing in positive outcomes tend to help create those outcomes as long as we are willing to put in the time and work.

In recovery we must make a choice: Are we walking away from the disease or toward the next crisis? It doesn't matter if it's a drink or drug or serious disease. I choose to journey outward, letting trouble shrink in the rear view, not ignored, but kept in its place. Later I will distill this concept into two types: the Fighters and the Waiters.

20 – Cancer Stinks

In joining the community of brain cancer patients, one finds people of all walks of life who are dealing with the uncertainty of the disease as well as the advancements of treatments. Early on I was introduced to Dr. Joe B and his son.

Joe is an orthopedic surgeon and Joe Jr. —I call him Mighty Joe Younger — is an active young man who was just about to turn 18. He is a soccer player and normal in most senses of the word except that he was diagnosed with GBM in the fall of 2012. Joe's symptoms were far more severe than mine. But his is also a positive story because of his overall attitude and the hard work and devotion of his family especially his father.

Dr. B has made a second career out of tracking the best information on GBM, both through traditional medicine and alternative approaches. He has focused on the basics: diet and exercise, which can make a world of difference. But he also looked at anything that can give his son a fighting chance. Both Joes have been inspirational to me and should be to anyone battling a serious illness.

Among the many resources Joe found was the writings of Dr. Ben Williams, a PhD in psychology and a man who has survived GBM since the mid 90's. He was diagnosed at age 50. Dr. Williams, unlike medically trained Dr. Joe, is an educated professional who is interested in saving his own life and helping those who are also faced with this persistent tumor. He has already beat the odds by years! When Ben was diagnosed few people survived GBM longer than a year, with most passing away within the first four months of the diagnosis. You can search his work. He has a 120 plus page treatise that spans 15 years of successfully beating this cancer. It is both impressive and sobering.

Dr. Joe also introduced me to Cheryl B. Her story is a fascinating one that spans more than a decade of survival, although at times difficult and included several surgeries. Cheryl and I have stayed in touch and she is positive, active and willing to try reasonable approaches to control her tumor. Cheryl's book is called Life's Mountains and is available on Amazon.com

At this point in a typical book about a specific disease – and there are many — the author might list some of the treatment options and success (or lack of) with each. I have decided not to do that and the reason is simple. The great majority of those reading this do not have GBM and probably will not have to deal with this brain tumor. If you do then I hope you are getting good medical care. My point is that of all those I have encountered on this journey there are two clear groups: the fighters and the waiters. You can see them in the holding area for radiation treatment, or in the infusion centers. This does not just apply to brain cancer but most cancers. The fighters are smiling and engaging others, they make eye contact and are willing to share their experiences while remaining as positive as they can. The waiters are usually quiet and sad except for complaints (most justifiable, but again does it really help?). The fighters often have companions who are just as upbeat and engaging. Sadly the waiters are often alone.

I would never presume to understand the plight of another, especially when I know the bleak horizon that might lie ahead. But giving in to the bad news and allowing that to frame our very existence is by definition a conclusion. For me there is never one ending. I have seen too many final chapters rewritten, I have rewritten many of them myself. While fighting and embracing life today may change nothing, it seems to be a better path and a better way to spend this moment.

Recently I witnessed a fighter transform into a waiter within a day. She was in the fight of her life and the treatments had become painful to the point of debilitating. The last thing she said to me was, "I quit."

"Please don't." I said, but the words echoed as hollow as a wood block in a kindergarten orchestra. She could not swallow and speaking was torture all due, she said, to the radiation treatments. A sinking feeling came over me. I wanted to believe she could work through this set back. But one never knows.

I am not sure if it's the chemo, or the part of my brain impacted by the tumor, the surgery, or the radiation treatments, but smells are intensified by a factor of ten and sensitivity to things that were mild irritants such as dairy prompted a higher reaction than before. And bad smells attack like a battalion of marines. Even things most people would think smell wonderful, such as toast or a bakery or fresh brewed coffee can trigger a bitter response. It's unpredictable and one of those little things that make my recovery unusual and sometimes difficult.

After five weeks of radiation and chemo therapy, Monika and I figured out a reasonable schedule of exercise, rest and foods that help me stay fairly comfortable. It was not easy to determine and it's much more complicated for most others.

Such is life in this weird existence, a phrase borrowed from an old friend Tom C. I wake up early, get the schedule started and try not to overdo or under do the things that are important. Eating is the biggest challenge. Most things simply don't taste very appealing, much like the smells, it is impossible to predict.

21 – "Hope I'm Funny"

Richard Pryor used to open every act with the following: "Hi, I'm Richard. Hope I'm funny." I never saw or heard Richard Pryor when he wasn't funny, near the end tragically, flawed and hopelessly funny. But he always met and exceeded that humble hope. His story if one of pulling comedy out of abject desperation and eventually desperation won. But did it? His body of work is not of a drug addict, burn victim or even infirmed, it is of a man who seldom worried about what others thought and presented his talents the best he could.

It is perhaps the most difficult thing any performer can do, ignore the reflection from the eyes of the audience and simply do your best. It is also not easy when the audience is unseen, such as a radio audience.

In 1974 I was still in awe of the fact that I worked at a radio station, surrounded by some of the most talented and best known stars of the medium. One day I was sitting in a control room watching Larry Morrow do his morning show. Larry was a genius communicator and practiced in the art of charming almost anyone. He made a mistake, it was a small one, perhaps no one would have guessed other than Larry and me, the young engineer. Later I asked Larry about the error. He said something I will never forget, "In all the years, all the hours I have been on the radio, and there have been many, I have never done a perfect airshift. It just doesn't exist."

This had a profound effect on me. Not just that he said it, but that he knew it up front and still worked day after day, minute after minute with no regard at all to the inevitable flaw waiting just ahead. He said something else, "isn't it funny how we only expect ourselves to be perfect, when in fact, nobody cares?"

Larry was right and it has been said in different ways a million times before. We sometimes tear ourselves apart concerned over what others think when the truth is the observer, whoever he or she might be, is only concerned with his own imperfection. I believe it is a great piston in the engine of human dynamics. And while it is truly a motivator, it can also act as a great drag on accomplishment.

22 – Terminal Tower

In the early Twentieth Century my town, Cleveland, Ohio, presented itself among the big boys; New York, Chicago, Philadelphia and Detroit. Known then as the Sixth City with a population that teetered around one million it was a rail and Lake Port for the heavy commerce. It had the tools and muscle, but lacked original vision. I think Cleveland still suffers from that today.

In 1930 there was a big hoopla in the center of town as the second tallest building in the nation was dedicated. A couple of odd brothers were anxious to show off their version of Grand Central Station with a tower New York could not manage to construct over their great rail terminal (so they put a huge edifice a few blocks away, the Empire State Building).

The Van Sweringen brothers made their fortunes on rail and real estate. They were among the Cleveland tycoons born of the industrial boom that had rippled around the world more than a century before. Their building was a triumph and still stands, often brightly lit over a resurgent downtown.

When I was a child I adored the marble and brass Art Deco interior of the train station, the personalities who gathered there and sounds and smells of the place. There was always odor of ozone and oxidizing iron from the trains and electric light rail lines that ran just beneath the floors, the diesel and even old coal-fired engines as they came in and loaded onto an amazing "turning platform" for a slow 180 degree spin before departing. The heavy notes from below were joined in a sensory soup of roasting peanuts, coffee and caramel popcorn from the ornate kiosk and sometimes steaks in the restaurants along the concourse.

Men in hats and women in furs stepped casually, but purposefully to and from the shops and ultimately to their train platforms. We were, to them, part of the backdrop, a young colored family with a curious little boy whose stare might have added to their air of propriety. It was my secret. I was that happy little boy, and I could see on most of their faces that they probably carried too large a burden, too much self importance to know that feeling often or for very long.

Sometimes the shine man would gesture with blackened fingers clutching a dime to come over to his stand. With a wink he would ask, "tell me what that fellow does for a living," he would tip his chin upward at a passing stranger, "and this mercury lady is yours!" I would say insurance salesman! The shine man would drop the dime in my hand. It was a little game we played. They were all insurance salesmen. My dad would laugh, "got him again, did you sonny?"

"Yep Pop. But I think he knows."

"I think so, too. It's not what a man does for a living, it's how he lives."

The shine man was also happy.

That tower stood at the end of our bus rides down Euclid or Superior, getting bigger as we closed in on whatever extended errands would draw us downtown. It was exhilarating until one day, when I heard the word, the hallowed name of that wonderful and personal Emerald City in a different context.

If ever my mother had a closer friend than her oldest sister she never let on. Aunt Lena was stunningly hilarious and seemed totally fearless. She could drink her baby brother, Wayman under the table and make mom and dad laugh so hard I often worried about their well being. Lena looked enough like my mom to be very attractive to me, but by the time we were around Aunt Lena her only child had already grown up and joined the navy. She was pretty much done with kids. It was okay, I loved her anyway.

'Terminal lung cancer,' were probably the three saddest words I had heard from my mom to that point as she ended the phone call with her beloved sister. I don't know if I have ever heard sadder words from my mother until my father's death in 1986.

Now my tower's first name had a new, painful and honestly silly connotation. Why would anyone give such a beautiful and vibrant place a name related to *death*?

Of course terminals can be starting places as easily as endings, arrivals as well as departures. But I began calling the tower the Gateway – and later in life it became "Poppy's Tower." But that's another story for the next volume. Oddly enough, many years later that name became associated with an entertainment complex that included a new stadium for the Cleveland Indians and a multipurpose arena that was home for the Cleveland Cavaliers.

Words do have meaning, and although the medical field has all but abandoned use of the word "terminal," it still exists. In every way we are all terminal. 'Stage four' seems to have replaced terminal to describe the finality of certain diseases, but even that has a little wiggle room. There are several stories featured in this book and many more that defuse the hopelessness of both terms.

My form of brain tumor might have those terrible tags, but there is another thing I've learned about words: They only mean what they are fed. All the words in the universe, all the adverse definitions of things real and imagined cannot stand up to the power of attitude and intention.

I really believe we are more than that, more than words and certainly more than diseases that might come our way.

Perhaps much more.

23 – Bird Tree

We are fortunate enough to have 30 or 40 trees standing tall around our nearly acre of property.

In spring every tree is filled with the sights and sounds of cardinals, colorful little Carolina chickadees, blue jays, robins and much more. In each tree renewed life bursts in fluttering wings and cheerful songs.

It should come as no surprise that I met a man, a physician whose surname translates from original German to English as "bird tree."

This chapter is about Dr. Vogelbaum and the Cleveland Clinic. But it's much more than that. It's about a renewal, a change and a chance. It started by taking the recommendation from our Summa oncologist to seek a second opinion. We had both University Hospitals and Cleveland Clinic in our network, two of the finest medical and research institutions in the world and both within 45 minutes of our home. Dr. Mahesh had worked with one oncologist at the Rose Ella Burkhardt Brain Tumor and Neuro-Oncology Center at the Cleveland Clinic. Before that moment I was less inclined to pursue any other opinions. But I got a clear sense that there was more that could be done. And there was. After a series of examinations and conversations at Cleveland Clinic we sat face to face with Dr. Michael Vogelbaum.

By his own words, he took my case not because it was easy, but because it was challenging and the one intangible that he and I, and I hope that by now you believe, too, was abundantly present. That is a positive attitude and every intention to win.

Damn the odds.

Just days prior to this fateful conversation with Dr. Mahesh I spoke to a dear friend who had lost his wife to cancer three years prior. In talking about his experience he mentioned that his beloved wife decided not to have a second opinion. While I respect that, I also found it profound on many levels.

Second opinions are standard and the more dire the outlook the more important that additional information becomes.

As discussed earlier, those of us in Northeast Ohio are lucky for many reasons. Growing up in Cleveland there were a few gems in an otherwise rusting bracelet wrapping the northeast corner of the Midwest. The Cleveland Orchestra guided by the genius of George Szell, one of the greatest conductors of the 20th Century, was considered among the world's most accomplished and sought after performing arts institutions — some would argue that it still is. The Cleveland Museum of Art housed some of the most famous and compelling collections on the globe. These two entities alone kept my town from sliding into the Cuyahoga River, merely a footnote in America's industrial decline. It was not easy. Most of the city did fade into a pathos that was painful and self-inflicted.

In the 1920's things were quite different. The Cleveland Indians won the World Series. A year later three doctors who had experienced the challenges at the dawn of modern medicine in the most unforgiving of classrooms: the trenches and hedgerows of WWI-torn Europe came home. Drs. Frank Emory Bunts, George Washington Crile, and William Edgar Lower, developed a new kind of hospital. The idea was simple, why not gather doctors of different disciplines and focus their knowledge and expertise on one disease and in some cases one patient?

Today that interdisciplinary approach is the standard where budgets and research can attract the kind of talent necessary. And it has made Cleveland Clinic one of the top medical facilities in the world. On staff at the neurooncology institute is the distinguished Dr. Michael Vogelbaum.

It is important to note here that what will follow is by no means a reflection, critical or otherwise, of the care and treatment I received at our (Summa) brain health facility or the neurosurgeons and their team who performed at exemplary levels. This has been reinforced at every level of this journey including at Cleveland Clinic. Summa's Cooper Cancer Center may be smaller, but we are extremely fortunate to have these talented and dedicate men and women ready and able to perform miracles. But they understand that within an hour's drive and within the ample network set up by this innovative system, they can tap the knowledge and technology of the world's best.

24 – The Crystal Cave and The Sight

In 1970 Mary Stewart began publishing a wonderful series of books about Merlin the Wizard and his magical origins. The mythical man was given little back story until then. The great adventures were left to King Arthur, his most famous student.

But the Wizard did have an origin, and in Mary Stewart's imagination it was rich with memorable characters, struggles and heroism.

In the Crystal Cave, where Merlin was conceived, the forces began to divide, take sides and do battle. Instability resulted from greed and the great prize was the "Gift of Sight." Let's call it *truth*.

Sight was the ability to see past, present, future and in some cases hidden realities that can portend dangerous consequences. When you examine stories like these, whether it is Lord of the Rings, Chronicles of Narnia, Harry Potter or any epic fantasy adventure, it all comes down to clear, honest vision and removing the veil that seems to surround much of life's biggest secrets. If you have an adventurous pre-teen or restless adolescence, I highly recommend Ms Stewart's work. I am not surprised it was overlooked by Hollywood. It is an experience that is best enjoyed in its written form.

Modern wizards, real wizards are among us. And while I will resist adding magical powers to the humans who have worked so hard to save my life and the lives of so many, I will acknowledge that what they do is extraordinary. I define imagination as the one ability by which humans can claim superiority over the world. It is not too far of a reach to see parallels in the story of Merlin and the career of Dr. Vogelbaum and those like him. I suspect he might find this a bit of an over-reach.

With the help of Dr. Vogelbaum and others, Cleveland Clinic has created a special operating theatre that allows magnetic resonance imaging (MRI) in near real-time during the procedure. Within minutes of the surgeons working inside the brain they saw actual images of the tumor. He also used a special dye that illuminates the malignancy so that he can see and remove as much as safely possible. This is a simplification of a very complex procedure. The end result should be a much smaller mass, thus less work for the radiation and chemotherapy. It is all about seeing the unseen.

Dr. Vogelbaum was perhaps the most fascinating of the exceptional men and women I had encountered along the way. That is not to diminish those we have met thus far, but there was something deep in his gray eyes and modest smile that said: "we can do this! We will do this."

On Wednesday, August 28th, Poppy's 33rd birthday — and I am grateful that she was there with Monika — Dr. Vogelbaum and his team at Cleveland Clinic entered my skull armed with the 2013 version of

The Sight. There was every expectation that I would come out at least as well as the first surgery; that I will be able to continue not only with this work but the next edition. And that I will finish the next novel in the Radio Murders Series titled "Barbicas."

And so it is true. Five days later and this chapter has been added. While the fiction writer in me can't help but find deeper symbolism and a literary narrative in what has happened to us, the facts are these: I have a chance to turn a potential tragedy into a beam of hope for those who are fighting an awful darkness. Imagine not knowing what is real, not recognizing those you love and being unsure of the sights and sounds that should be second nature and easily recognized. Imagine the words cancer and brain tumor becoming so ingrained in your identity that they almost replace your name in a waiting room. Then imagine your life compressed into a time frame that is not only shortened, but possibly already limited to a date circled on a calendar. These are stark new realities faced by tens of thousands every day. But before those impressions take hold, there is an alternate way of viewing this reality that, I believe, can make all the difference in the world.

It starts like this: "I am not going to let this control me. I am going to control it!" Then recruit the army to make it happen!

Part of that army are the right doctors and treatment options. I have mentioned many of those doctors already, but as I was working on a late draft of this book I asked one of my favorite oncologist if I could use his name. He said that it would probably be okay but he wanted to discuss it with me in private first. After I showed him the passages where he is featured he agreed to openly participate in the story. His concern was that I might be ascribing too much power to the science and the scientists to overcome cancer. I certainly hope I am not giving you that impression.

Monika and I have met some dedicated people providing a fighting chance to hundreds of patience. But this fight is far from over. Each has special tools and talents and together they form a strong line of defense, but the dragon is still there, still breathing fire and taking far too many of us out of this life. My purpose is to reinforce how we can and must join the battle by doing the things to stay strong, physically and mentally. To do otherwise, for me, is unthinkable!

RoBBing Mind

To Be Continued
Randy and Yul

From the time I was a child and after more than 40 years a media professional, I have been fascinated by the power certain people attained after death. Abraham Lincoln, John F. Kennedy, Ronald Reagan, entertainment personalities Elvis Presley, Jimi Hendrix and many more gained greater prominence postmortem. And there are others who took the phenomenon even further by planning to deliver a specific message from beyond the grave.

This small book is the result of a focused desire to track the possibilities, good and bad, as surgeons and others discovered and attacked a cancer growing in my brain. This journal began from the start of this journey for two reasons, firstly, to add an intimate perspective to a serious brain health event, one many have and might face. And secondly I wanted to know — as soon as possible — if I was losing capabilities, if I was being robbed of my mind, and for me there is no quicker indication than the inability to write with clarity.

I must admit that while I worked hard on this book throughout the experience, prescribed steroids and other changes in perception made the original work messy, to be kind, and it took the help of my friend and editor Pat Fernberg as well as others and a

125

good deal of additional time before we were able to cobble together a work worthy of your time and hopefully your recommendation.

There is no doubt that I am extremely fortunate. And to those who are reading this perhaps because my good fortune simply wasn't there for you or time is running out, I cannot express enough my wishes that things were different. But I have seen miracles in abundance. Therapies have improved beyond anyone's wildest expectation. The brain itself, being such a remarkable organism, finds ways to re-route, reassign and even rebuild abilities.

Carnegie Mellon University professor Randy Pausch was handed a timetable in 2006 by cancer doctors. His disease, pancreatic cancer, was faster, more invasive, and far deadlier than mine. He made the most of his last days, creating as his legacy a highly prized series of talks, The Last Lecture: Achieving Your Childhood Dreams, that will inform and enlighten generations to come. His was not a wasted life, nor a death in vain.

In the mid-eighties Yul Brynner, who enjoyed a long career playing some of the most memorable roles ever seen on stage and screen, learned that he had lung cancer. Mr. Brynner concluded that it had been caused by years of cigarette smoking. The day after he passed away, a startling commercial began appearing on TV featuring a gaunt man who barely resembled the King of Siam or the Pharaoh Ramses II.

In it, Mr. Brynner made it clear that he was now dead, and it is because he smoked. He pleaded with the viewer to quit: "Quit now before you end up like me." I suspect he changed a lot of minds and, in doing so, saved a lot of lives.

Monika and I have thought, talked and prayed a lot about this adventure, and it always comes back to this: We can live or not. We could get T-boned on Route 91 or, as was almost the case several years ago, or a gas leak could send our dream house — and us — into oblivion in an instant.

For now, extraordinary therapies are working. I have a fine team here in Akron at Summa and at Cleveland Clinic. One person I need to mention is Dr. Chirag Shah, my radiation-oncologist. He works in concert with Dr. Mahesh and the two are an amazing team, along with the technologists handling the machines. They are accomplished scientist and medical practitioners, but they are also partners in my recovery and that is priceless.

For now, I am fine and I have a lot of work to do. I don't see that changing anytime soon. The doctors, nurses, med techs, hospital workers in every role, volunteers, researchers, and my family and friends are not giving up. It is not in their nature, and it certainly is not in the DNA of Monika and Chuck. With so much love and energy there is only one possible outcome. It looks very bright, very bright indeed.

If you go on Amazon or visit your local book store you will find a large number of books written by people diagnosed with various types and stages of cancer. Many are very good and enlightening. But most, I am convinced were conceived out of a touch of desperation and the need to leave something should the disease win. Sometimes writing is used to stem the boredom of a long-term recovery in which one cannot return to normal work. For me writing is part of my work and this fits right in.

The beauty of this gift I have been given is that the more you share the greater it becomes and the greater value it is to the recipients. Of that there is no doubt at all. So here is just the beginning of sharing possibilities, recovery and healing. I can only hope it helps someone.

Please pass it along.

RoBBing Mind

Acknowledgements and

Thanks

None of this would be possible without the help, love and encouragement of some very special people and institutions

Summa Health System, Akron Ohio

The Cleveland Clinic

All the medical professionals and support staff who have dedicated their lives to helping people get and stay well;

Tony and Diane Agnesi

The D. Wallace Family; Dr. Franciska Kiraly

The Rubber City Radio Group: My Professional Family, all; especially Thom Mandel, Joyce Lagios, Mark Biviano, Ray Horner, Kathy Pearson, Teri Jones, Tim Daugherty, Sue Wilson and Edward Esposito

My family Poppy Coleman and Monika

My Sister Barbara Binder, Vykki and her children

The Polks, Jacksons, Kings, Bibbs and Parkers, Monika's sister Cecilia; Lou Lange;

Daniel Steinberg – who has known the ultimate heart break, yet soldiers on.

And a very special thanks and eternal gratitude for

Dr. Terry Gordon,

a man who has known life's greatest accomplishments, wonders and tragedies, yet still walks this spiritual journey in a way that is truly inspirational!

About Chuck

Chuck Collins is a 40-year veteran of broadcasting and media in Northeast Ohio, most recently in Akron, Ohio. He is currently operations director with Rubber City Radio Group, WAKR, WQMX, WONE, and has been on the WAKR air 10-3pm weekdays for the last 7 years.

Chuck has written four novels and published hundreds of essays for online and other publications. He has supported the performing arts with leadership roles in the Greater Akron Musical Association and continues to work with alcoholics and recovery services as a trustee with IBH, Addiction Recovery Center.

Chuck and his wife Monika are devoted to family and community and live in Hudson, Ohio.

Good treatment and a good attitude will help me produce Robbing Mind 2: Recovery.

Personal note: You will wake up some mornings in a fog of doubt. You will feel more and more irrelevant and wonder why fight one more day? When that happens, please remember this, even before you became ill, all you had was one day. But this day is special and it will not be complete until you add your spirit to it.

Eat, move around, see the spark of life, of the divine in the smallest things, do what you can and this day will reward you with another just like it, only better!

Chuck Collins